THE UNEART
OF ACTIVATI
CLE.......

A Step-By-Step Guide To Leveraging The Benefits Of Activated Charcoal For A Safe And Effective Detoxification

MURPHY KENNETH

1

Contents

CHAPTER ONE
Introduction

In order to make a highly porous substance with a large surface area, oxygen is used to treat carbon, resulting in activated charcoal.

This enables it to eliminate poisons, chemicals, and gases from the body by binding to them in the digestive tract. Charcoal's adsorption characteristics are enhanced through the activation process, which entails heating the material to high temperatures, so creating millions of microscopic pores and fissures on the surface.

Uses For Activated Charcoal

• Activated charcoal has many applications, one of which is as a detoxifying agent. It aids in the detoxification process by binding to and removing toxins, heavy metals, and other toxic chemicals.

• Activated charcoal's ability to bind to gas and other chemicals in the digestive tract has been linked to improved digestive health symptoms like bloating and flatulence.

• Activated charcoal is a common component of all-natural tooth pastes and other teeth whitening solutions. It is thought to help whiten teeth by attracting and soaking up discoloration and debris on the teeth.

• Activated charcoal can be used in face masks and other skincare products to draw out impurities and clean the skin.

• Activated charcoal's antioxidant qualities have been studied for their potential anti-aging benefits by neutralizing free radicals before they may cause cell and tissue damage.

While activated charcoal may help with some conditions, it is not a panacea and should not be taken in place of professional medical care. It should also be taken separately from other vitamins and drugs because it can inhibit their absorption. You should always check with your doctor before trying out a new substance, including activated charcoal.

An Explanation Of What An Activated Charcoal Bath Is And How It Helps

Consuming activated charcoal as part of a detox program is a popular new approach to cleansing the body of harmful chemicals and heavy metals.

In order to make a highly porous substance with a large surface area, oxygen is used to treat carbon, resulting in activated charcoal. This enables it to eliminate poisons, chemicals, and gases from the body by binding to them in the digestive tract.

Activated charcoal can be used in the form of capsules, pills, powder, or liquid during a cleanse. After entering the stomach, the activated charcoal travels through the digestive tract, where it absorbs harmful substances before being expelled from the body in the form of feces.

Supporters of activated charcoal cleanse say it can enhance general health by flushing out toxins and is particularly effective for digestive ailments including bloating, gas, and diarrhea. However, the efficacy of activated charcoal cleansing is still debatable, and there is only a little amount of research to back up these claims.

While activated charcoal has a high safety profile, it is best to take it on its own rather than with other supplements or drugs to avoid any possible interactions. Constipation or black stools, while worrisome, are usually not harmful effects.

CHAPTER TWO
Cleansing Preparation

Make sure it is safe for you to do so by checking with your doctor before beginning an activated charcoal cleanse. It is recommended to see a doctor before using activated charcoal due to possible drug interactions.

If your doctor has given you the go-ahead, here are some things you should know before beginning an activated charcoal cleanse:

• Get enough of fluids: Activated charcoal can lead to dehydration, therefore it is crucial to replenish lost fluids before, during, and after the cleanse.

• Consume a diet high in fiber and low in processed foods in the days leading up to the cleanse. This will help you get ready for the cleanse by ensuring that your digestive system is in top shape.

• Caffeine and alcohol can both reduce the efficiency of the activated charcoal, therefore it is recommended to abstain from both for a while before beginning the cleanse.

• If you have never used activated charcoal before, it is best to ease into it by starting with a low dose and working your way up. Any negative effects can be lessened in this way.

• Taking a probiotic supplement during and after a cleanse can help to restore beneficial microorganisms that may be lost due to the use of activated charcoal.

Never mistake a detox for a permanent solution to your health problems. In order to keep feeling healthy and strong, it is crucial to stick to a routine of healthy eating and physical activity.

How To Cleanse Properly With Detailed Step-By-Step Guide

Because of its effectiveness at binding to toxins and impurities in the digestive tract, activated charcoal is frequently used for cleansing reasons. Follow these simple steps for a deep cleansing using activated charcoal:

• Time it right: Because this cleanse may have some short-term adverse effects, it is best to do it when you will not have any pressing obligations or engagements.

• You may get activated charcoal capsules from a pharmacy or a health food store. Verify that the pills contain only activated charcoal and nothing else.

• Take two or three capsules of activated charcoal with a full glass of water first thing in the morning.

Do this for three days in a row, three or four times each day.

• To aid in the elimination of harmful substances, up your water consumption to at least 10 glasses daily.

• Solid food should be avoided as much as possible during the cleansing process. Instead, try supporting your body's detoxification process with homemade vegetable juices or bone broth.

• Stop doing the activated charcoal cleanse for at least two weeks after the first three days if you can help it.

Warning: If you are on any prescription drugs, you should talk to your doctor before beginning this cleanse since activated charcoal may interact with them. People who are pregnant or nursing, or who have a history of digestive issues, should also avoid this cleanse.

CHAPTER THREE
Supplements With Activated Charcoal: When To Take Them

The suggested time between doses of activated charcoal supplements varies from person to person and treatment goal. Some broad rules of thumb are as follows:

• Activated charcoal supplements, taken with a full glass of water 30 minutes before meals, can aid digestion. Gas, bloating, and other digestive problems may be alleviated as a result.

• Detoxification can be aided by taking activated charcoal capsules either two hours before or after a meal. Do this twice or thrice a day for up to a week.

• Activated charcoal pills should be taken daily, once before or after eating, for optimal health.

You should talk to your doctor before beginning any supplement routine, as activated charcoal may reduce the effectiveness of several drugs. To prevent dehydration, take activated charcoal with plenty of water, and keep in mind that its prolonged usage can cause nutritional deficiencies.

Supplementing Your Charcoal Cleanse With Other Detox Methods

In addition to a charcoal cleanse, there are a number of other detoxification methods you might try. Consider these alternates:

• Keep your body hydrated; doing so will aid in the elimination of harmful substances. Keep your body hydrated and free of toxins by drinking at least eight glasses of water daily.

• Consume a diet high in fruits and vegetables; they are excellent sources of detoxifying nutrients like vitamins, minerals, and antioxidants. Leafy greens, berries, citrus fruits, and cruciferous veggies like broccoli and cauliflower are all excellent choices.

• The lymphatic system, which is in charge of flushing out harmful pollutants, can be stimulated with regular exercise. Walk, jog, or ride a bike at a moderate pace for at least 30 minutes per day.

• Do some deep breathing exercises or try meditation to lower your stress levels and help your body eliminate toxins more efficiently.

• Try dry brushing, which entails gently exfoliating the skin with a dry brush while also stimulating the lymphatic system. This may aid in detoxification and vascular health.

• Think about using a sauna or steam room: these facilities are great for helping you sweat off toxins through increased perspiration.

While these methods may help facilitate your body's natural detoxification mechanisms, they are not intended to replace professional medical care or advice. Consult a medical expert before beginning any detoxification program or if you have any health concerns.

Post-Cleanse

Post-cleanse is the time after a fast, detox, or other dietary procedure has been completed. Reintroducing foods should be done slowly and carefully during this time to prevent gastrointestinal discomfort and other potential health problems.

Think about the following as you make the shift back to a normal eating routine:

• Light, easily digested foods like soups, steamed vegetables, and fruits should be your first course.

• Stay away from things like refined sugars and artificial additives, as well as processed and fried foods.

• Drink plenty of water, herbal teas, and fresh juices to keep your body hydrated.

• Eat more probiotic-rich foods like yogurt, kimchi, and sauerkraut to encourage good bacteria in the digestive tract.

• Keep track of how your body reacts to each new food, and work your way back up to heavier and more complex fare.

• Respect your body and give it time to heal. Give yourself some time to readjust and develop a routine that works for you.

Keep in mind that a cleanse or detox is just a short-term method of assisting your body's own cleansing mechanisms. Long-term success depends on sticking to a nutritious eating plan.

CHAPTER FOUR
How To Deal With Charcoal Cleanse Complications

Consuming activated charcoal to remove toxins and impurities from the body is a common detox procedure known as a charcoal cleanse or activated charcoal cleanse.

Some people may find it helpful, but there are risks you should be aware of. Some of the most common ones, and how to deal with them, are as follows.

• Because it soaks up liquid and slows down digestion, activated charcoal can lead to the unpleasant side effect of constipation. Fiber supplements and plenty of water can help with this.

• Activated charcoal may have the reverse effect and produce diarrhea in certain people. To cope with this, cut back on the amount of charcoal you eat and drink more water.

• Some people on a charcoal detox report feeling sick to their stomachs and throwing up. Stop taking the charcoal and instead try some ginger tea or ginger pills if you are feeling nauseous.

• In some people, taking activated charcoal might lead to cramping in the stomach. Reduce your charcoal intake and alleviate the discomfort with a heating pad or a hot bath.

• Some drugs, such as birth control pills and antidepressants, may be less effective when taken with activated charcoal because it reduces their absorption. Before beginning a charcoal cleanse, it is recommended that you consult your doctor.

Keep in mind that a charcoal cleanse is not for everyone and should not be done regularly. Stop the cleanse and visit a doctor if you have any serious or ongoing negative effects.

Meal And Snack Ideas For The Charcoal Cleanse

Consume nutrient-dense foods and stay away from processed and junk food when on a charcoal cleanse. Healthy, flavorful, and suitable for a charcoal cleanse, here are some sample recipes for meals and snacks:

1. Bowl of charcoal smoothies:

• Banana, one, frozen.

• One-half cup of frozen berries.

• (1) Half a cup of almond milk.

• 1 tablespoon of activated charcoal.

• Banana slices, berries, coconut flakes, and granola make great toppings.

Mix the activated charcoal powder, almond milk, banana, and berries in a blender until smooth. Place in a bowl and garnish with fruit, coconut, granola, and banana slices.

2. Salad with quinoa and vegetables:

• One cup of quinoa, cooked.

• Cucumber, about 1/2 cup chopped.

• 12 cup of finely sliced bell pepper.

• Fifty grams of fresh, chopped basil.

• Chopped fresh parsley, 2 tablespoons

• 1 tablespoon olive oil.

• Lemon juice, 1 tablespoon.

• The right amount of salt and pepper.

Toss the quinoa with the bell pepper, cucumber, cherry tomatoes, and parsley. Season with salt and pepper and drizzle with olive oil and lemon juice.

3. Sweet potato fries, baked

• 2 sweet potatoes, medium.

- Coconut oil, 1 tablespoon.

- Smoked paprika, 1 teaspoon.

- Garlic powder, 1 teaspoon.

- The right amount of salt and pepper.

Start by setting your oven temperature to 400 degrees Fahrenheit. Prepare the sweet potatoes as directed, frying them in coconut oil and seasoning them with smoky paprika, garlic powder, salt, and pepper. Bake the fries in a single layer for 20-25 minutes, or until they reach the desired crispiness.

4. Hummus with Charcoal:

• 1 can chickpeas, drained and rinsed.

• 2 Tablespoons Tahini.

• Lemon juice, 2 tablespoons.

• 1 minced clove of garlic.

• 1 tablespoon olive oil.

• 1 tablespoon of activated charcoal.

• The right amount of salt and pepper.

Make a smooth paste in a food processor by combining chickpeas, tahini, lemon juice, garlic, olive oil, and activated charcoal powder. Put in as much salt and pepper as you like.

During a charcoal cleanse, it is important to pay attention to your body and eat what it requires.

CHAPTER FIVE
A Review Of The Pros And Cons Of An Activated Charcoal Detoxification

Consuming activated charcoal as part of a cleanse is a common way to get rid of harmful substances from the body. The advantages and disadvantages of this approach are briefly reviewed below.

Benefits:

• Possible benefit in alleviating gas and bloating.

• Possible benefit to skin health.

• Food poisoning symptoms may be relieved.

• Potentially beneficial for kidney and liver health.

• Possible aid in gastrointestinal health and inflammation reduction.

Negative Implications:

• Could lead to tummy troubles or loose stools.

• The potential for sickness is present.

• It may decrease drug absorption, for example.

• Long-term consumption may cause nutritional deficits.

• Potential incompatibility with specific medical conditions.

Despite its potential usefulness, activated charcoal should not be used in place of conventional medical care or a healthy lifestyle. Before beginning any kind of diet or detox program, it is best to talk to a doctor.

Conclusions And Suggestions

In conclusion, some people may find relief from bloating and enhancement of skin health after doing a charcoal cleanse.

Constipation, diarrhea, and decreased medicine absorption are only few of the possible negative side effects. Activated charcoal should be avoided for the long-term since it can cause nutritional deficits.

It is worth noting that a charcoal cleanse has not been thoroughly studied in the scientific community.

In addition, before beginning a detox or nutrition program, it is crucial to speak with a healthcare practitioner if you have any preexisting health concerns.

Eat plenty of nutrient-dense foods, drink enough of water, and pay attention to your body if you decide to try a charcoal cleanse. Activated charcoal should be used sparingly and not combined with any other drugs or supplements.

The greatest way to maintain good health is to eat right, exercise frequently, drink enough of water, and get plenty of shut-eye each night. Seek the advice of a medical expert if you have questions about your health or are experiencing any symptoms that seem out of the ordinary.

THE END

Printed in Great Britain
by Amazon

33640092R00030